Obesity and Computer Use

What You Need to Know

By

Adetutu Ijose

Published By:

Jointheirs Publishing

JP

Obesity and Computer Use
What You Need to Know

Copyright © 2012

Jointheirs Publishing
Jointheirs Activities Incorporated
www.jointheirspublishing.com

ISBN – 1-46993-322-5

EAN – 978-1-46993-322-1

Printed in the United States of America

Obesity and Computer Use:

What You Need to Know

An Important Caution

The advice given in *Obesity and Computer Use: What You Need to Know* is based on an understanding of the effects of computer use on human behavior gained when I suffered life-threatening consequences of computer use that could not be effectively diagnosed or treated by conventional medical science.

I am not obese hence I have extended my understanding of the effect of computer use on the body's processes to what causes obesity.

For example, sedentary activity is a cause for weight gain and so because computer use is sedentary and many people stay on it for hours on end, It is obviously a recipe for weight gain and obesity.

An already obese person who becomes so engaged in computer use that he or she spends most of everyday in front of the computer has no hope of losing weight or reversing their obesity.

Consequently, computer use affects both the cause and the solution for obesity. It enhances the potential for obesity while reducing the chance for a reversal of the condition.

There are many other ways in which computer use contributes to obesity and they are discussed in this book.

I have written this book because the contribution of computer use to obesity is never considered when the topic is discussed in public and it seems everyone is in deliberate denial.

In a world that has become computer use dependent, ignoring computer use contributions is not an option if we are serious about reversing the trend.

All is not yet lost and this book aims to provide everyone with the information they need to make informed decisions on evaluating the contribution of computer use to any weight problem they may be having.

This book does not replace the advice of your medical doctors who knows you personally.

Please discuss any insight you gain from this book with your doctor before embarking on any of the suggested solutions or preventive actions.

I was able to get an understanding of my computer use induced health problems and identify the solution by gaining an understanding of the human code of existence from studying the human machine user manual we call the Bible or Scriptures.

Upon realizing I needed to be able to help others, I searched scientific text from all over the world in a bid to provide these insights to everyone else in a language they can understand.

These everyday presentations are what I have been providing for everyone in my various writings.

My book *Lessons I Learned the hard way: How to Identify Minimize Treat and Manage Computer Related Health Conditions* a 300 page guide on the subject of Computer use induced health conditions and the sequel *Computer Related Health Conditions: Understanding the Human Computer* contain many of these citations. If you want specific citations or additional information, please get a hold of these two books

If you are under treatment for any computer use induced health condition or if you suspect you might need such care, you must discuss any insight you gain from this book with your doctor before starting.

Please read the entire book carefully and help yourself and all you know. You must first acknowledge the need to do something. All the solutions are natural, cheap and do not involve medication.

In fact medicine is stressful to the body and one that is already weakened from the health effects of computer use should not be medicated. That will increase the stress and start new problems involving unnecessary costs that could bankrupt individuals, society as a nation and even globally.

We therefore need to change the way we have been looking at this issue if we want to remain a healthy prosperous population on earth.

One thing though, you must not self diagnose. Just look for a doctor who is ready to use other measures apart from medication as you will need close monitoring and some tests to identify what is depleted or missing in your body's system as a result of your computer use. These tests do not show everything but are a good starting point.

Computers are here to stay and can never be as safe as claimed. The computer use environment for example makes us look directly at a source of light to read, which is contrary to our natural way of never looking directly at the sun (our natural coded source of reading light).

It is always important to remember that the human body is a coded machine i.e. a living computer and like every other computer will have a problem when systems or software not coded with it are introduced to complement or replace its coded system.

Table of Contents

Chapter 1
What is Obesity

According to the National Library of Medicine – Pubmed Health[1-1], Obesity means having too much body fat.

The article stresses that it is not the same as being overweight, which means weighing too much. A person may be overweight from extra muscle, bone, or water, as well as from having too much fat.

Both terms however mean that a person's weight is higher than what is thought to be healthy for his or her height.

Body Mass Index (BMI)
According to The World Health Organization (WHO) Child Growth Standards Report[1-1], the Body mass index is the ratio - *weight (in kg)/recumbentt length or standing height (in m2).*

There are simpler ways of describing this ratio some of which we will find within this chapter.

For now let's start with a brief history of how the terminology BMI came to be and how it was derived.

In 1993 the WHO undertook a comprehensive review of the uses and interpretation of anthropometric references.

The review concluded that the NCHS/WHO growth reference, which had been recommended for international use since the late 1970s, did not adequately represent early childhood growth and that new growth curves were necessary.

The World Health Assembly endorsed this recommendation in 1994.

And between 1997 and 2003, WHO undertook the Multicentre Growth Reference Study (MGRS) to generate new curves for assessing the growth and development of children the world over.

Their report resulted in the first set of WHO Child Growth Standards (i.e. length/height-for-age, weight-for-age, weight-for-length, weight-for-height and body mass index (BMI)-for-age)

They came up with percentile and something called z-score curves for length/height-for-age, weight-for-age, weight-for-length, weight- for-height and BMI-for-age for boys and girls aged 0 to 60 months.

The National Institute of Health (NIH MEDPLUS) has a simple definition for BMI and how to measure it.

According to NIH MEDPLUS article on how to know your body Mass Index [1–2], BMI is a measure of body fat based on height and weight and it applies to children as well as adults both adult men and women.

The National Heart, Lung, and Blood Institute (NHLBI) has a Web site that lets you easily calculate your BMI just by entering your current height and weight. Visit www.nhlbisupport.com/bmi/bmicalc.htm to learn your BMI.

The NIH provides the following BMI categories

Underweight = <18.5

Normal weight = 18.5-24.9
Overweight = 25-29.9
Obesity = BMI of 30 or greater

Various other organizations have come up with various ways to carry out BMI assessment.

According to the NHLBI guidelines, assessment of overweight involves using three key measures:
1. Body mass index (BMI)

2. Waist circumference

3. Risk factors for diseases and conditions associated with obesity

BMI calculation has been made even simpler by the Centers for Disease Control and Prevention (CDC).

If you as an organization or an individual want to keep a tab on your BMI, it is possible to get a code you can cut and paste for a widget for the Adult BMI calculator for your website from the Centers for Disease Prevention and Control (CDC) website http://www.cdc.gov/obesity/

Worldwide BMI trends

According to the World Health Organization (WHO) [1-4], the BMI trends worldwide are as follows:
1. The prevalence of overweight and obesity were highest in the WHO Regions of the Americas (62% overweight in both sexes, and 26% for obesity)

2. They were lowest in the WHO Region for South East Asia (14% overweight in both sexes and 3% for obesity).

3. In the WHO Region for Europe and the WHO Region for the Eastern Mediterranean and the WHO Region for the Americas over 50% of women were overweight.

    For all three of these regions, roughly half of overweight women are obese (23% in Europe, 24% in the Eastern Mediterranean, 29% in the Americas).

    In all WHO regions women were more likely to be obese than men.

4. In the WHO regions for Africa, Eastern Mediterranean and South East Asia, women had roughly double the obesity prevalence of men

5. The prevalence of raised body mass index increases with income level of countries up to upper middle income levels.

6. The prevalence of overweight in high income and upper middle income countries was more than double that of low and lower middle income countries.

7. For obesity, the difference more than triples from 7% obesity in both sexes in lower middle income countries to 24% in upper middle income countries.

8. Women's obesity was significantly higher than men's, with the exception of high income countries where it was similar. In low and lower middle income countries, obesity among women was approximately double that among men.

Chapter 2
The Known Risk Factors for Obesity

Nobody likes to talk about the obvious cause of obesity –
our modern life and so called modern civilization.

But until we face the truth, accept it and begin to fit
ourselves into what is presented to us in the user manual
rather than trying to force a change that will never happen,
we will continue to suffer needlessly.

A code will always run in accordance with the process
coded. An attempt to put in extraneous activities or
processes will result in malfunction that will sooner than
later destroy the system. This is a factor we have all
realized from operating our computers.

This essentially means we as a generation of humans on the
earth are responsible for creating the obesity problems we
all complain about.

It will therefore take collective will to reverse the trend.

This realization is probably what gave rise to the let's
Move [2-1] initiative of Michelle Obama that depends on
collective action from everyone.

If you are a parent or anyone else involved with kids and
have not yet checked out this initiative, I will advise you to
do so.

Here are some of the many known risk factors in modern
day life responsible for today's obesity trends.

Low Physical Activity

A study on Trends over 5 Decades in U.S. Occupation-Related Physical Activity and Their Associations with obesity[2-2] said the folowing:

" in the early 1960s almost half the jobs in private industry in the US required at least moderate intensity activity whereas now less than 20% demand this level of energy expenditure"

They estimated that" for example, from 1960-62 to 2003-06, the occupation related daily energy expenditure decreased by 142 calories in men. They said the result was simillar for women.

It is safe to say that in this same period the population grew in terms of weight gain and obesity at a fast rate.

In fact, it is common knowledge known to most people by experience that weight gain is a natural consequence of a reduced energy expending activity lifestyle.

Since computer use falls into the category of low level energy expending activity its use will naturally be contributory to wieght gain and consequently obesity in its users especially those who have computer use dependent lifestyles.

Diet

This is a major factor in today's world with the high propensity that people have for eating fast food as well as processed and high fructose sugar containing food. In some parts of the USA, fried food is the staple. This is a major problem as this is a sure recipe for weight gain

In addition to all this, there is a tendency for people to go for the fast food when on the computer especially when trying to meet a deadline or just because the neurotransmitter depletions inherent in computer use affect the decision making abilities of every computer user.

Stress
Stress in a definite recipe for obesity especially when the body is overstressed beyond the limit coded for it. The user manual we call the Bible warns us about the adverse effect of stress essentially telling us we were coded to handle little stress i.e. just that inherent in carrying out normal body functions.

The kind of work and job functions that we have today are mostly not in agreement with the human body normal body system and so our everyday life in today's world is inherently overly stressful.

This explains why modern living absent of any other factor results in weight gain.

Our financial system including owning our homes by way of mortgage and the need to keep up with the Joneses, in addition results in a lot of financial worries. The manual admonishes us not to worry.

Many of the ways we operate today are not what we are coded for and consequently we are paying a high price for the so called "pleasures of life" that invariably create destruction in our body systems.

We may need to rethink our modern way of life, as it is definitely not working and the human system will never adjust, the manual makes that very plain.

We would be best served by retooling our modern lives to flow in accordance with the words of the manual so our bodies and we can be at peace with each other.

Cortisol
There is an article from the International Journal of Obesity [2-3] that links cortisol a hormone that is overproduced in the body in response to excessive stress to obesity.

Sleep Deprivation
Sleep time is when the body carries out most of its self repair work while the system is idling by design. It is the down time for daily repair necessitated by the wear and tear on the system from daily operating activities.

The human body just like any other machine does need daily down time to self repair.

With sleeplessness at epidemic proportions in the population, it is obvious we will definitely suffer a consequence from modern day lifestyles as sleeplessness results in stress and malfunction of the body's system.

Side Effect of Some Prescription Drugs
There are some drugs whose side effect is weight gain as they affect the various hormones and endocrine systems responsible for breaking down fat and other metabolic activities in the body.

Genetics
In some cases some people have a genetical predisposition to obesity and it could run in families.

It is not only what an individual is exposed to that matters. What their parents and other ancestors pass on to them is also important especially when still in the womb.

Consequently it is possible to be born with a predisposition for obesity.

Environmental Chemical and Light pollution
Here is a risk factor we all like to ignore but which I believe we cannot win the obesity war without addressing head on.

Industrialization has come at a high price and today's penchant for developing all kinds of synthetic chemicals not coded to operate in us in the name of research and corporate profit is nothing more than global human suicide.

We not only develop these chemicals, but introduce them into the food chain by way of genetical modification in the name of producing more food and feeding everyone.

What is the point of feeding everyone with poison. The user manual tells us how to farm and what we need to do to ensure bumper harvest. If we would use the manual we would be well served.

Today's culture is a culture of death and not of life. Many a times researchers tell us things will not hurt.

It is like throwing a virus into a computer system and saying it will not damage the system or the system will somehow magically change its code to accommodate the virus.

We all know that will never happen. It is the same with the human computer.

Finally, inherent in computer use is exposure to toxic chemicals and light fields that are stressful to our system. This is the subject matter of chapter 4.

Chapter 3
Childhood Obesity

According to Mayo Clinic[3-1], "Childhood obesity is a serious medical condition that affects children and adolescents. It occurs when a child is well above the normal weight for his or her age and height.

Childhood obesity is particularly troubling because the extra pounds often start children on the path to health problems that were once confined to adults, such as diabetes, high blood pressure and high cholesterol. Childhood obesity can also lead to poor self-esteem and depression.

One of the best strategies to reduce childhood obesity is to improve the diet and exercise habits of your entire family. Treating and preventing childhood obesity helps protect the health of your child now and in the future"

According to WebMD[3-2] Obese children are at risk for a number of conditions, including:
1. High cholesterol

2. High blood pressure

3. Early heart disease

4. Diabetes

5. Bone problems

6. Skin conditions such as heat rash, fungal infections, and acne

As we read in chapter 2, national focus has been brought to the issue of obesity in children by the Let's move initiative of Mrs. Obama in an attempt to bring everyone together as a national community to bring about a reversal in the current high level of obesity in American Chidren.

It would be great if all nations took an interest in developing simillar initiatives. It would drive down healthcare cost both now and in the future.

According to the WHO [3-2], BMI Cut-offs for children are as follows:

Age 5-19
Overweight: >+1SD (equivalent to BMI 25 kg/m^2 at 19 years)

Obesity: >+2SD
(equivalent to BMI 30 kg/m^2 at 19 years)

Thinness: <-2SD

Severe thinness: <-3SD

In 2006 the WHO [3-4] revised the growth standard for children to 5 years. There are about 30 standards. However only a few are routinely used one of which is the BMI

According to WHO Importantly, for the first time there now exist standardized Body Mass Index - BMI - charts for infants to age five, which is particularly useful for monitoring the increasing epidemic of childhood obesity.

In 2007 a change was made [3-5]. The BMI chart was merged with information from growth standard tables adopted by WHO in 1977 to come up with the new BMI charts for age 5 to 19. This was further tweaked in 1993 as we read in chapter 1 while discussing the general concept of BMI.

Chapter 4
Where Computer Use Comes in

The Sedentary nature of computer use

In their News Release dated 25 May 2011 [4-1], the Pennington Biomedical Research Center, said scientists found in a new study conducted that the decrease in workplace physical activity over the past fifty years is a significant contributor to the obesity epidemic.

The study they said suggests that changes in caloric intake cannot solely account for observed trends in weight gain increases for men and women in the United States

Computer use is virtually unavoidable in today's high tech world as we all go from desktops, laptops and, notebooks to cell phones, blackberries and iphones to kindle, ipads and other ereaders all day.

Some of us spend the most part of each day on computer devices and half of that time on the Internet browsing or chatting on social websites.

Then there are the many stories of marriages and jobs becoming unraveled as a result of sexting, texting Internet sexual activities and other issues that suggest people are becoming unhinged and our ability to maintain self-control is at risk.

For far too many of us our social life has become computer dependent and we may actually have become averse to anything that does not involve the computer and are kind of enslaved to it without consciously intending to or realizing we have come to that level of dependency

Many of our lives would be boring and uneventful without what we do on the Internet.

It all seems so convenient and harmless but is it? Are our brains and hearts sending the correct messages with regards to what is going on in our bodies or are we slowly deteriorating without knowing it.

Are our nerve receptors and sensors being infected or are they functioning properly?

It may also seem rather uncanny that so many new health issues seem to be popping up that conventional medicine seem unable to resolve and many biochemically related health issues are on the rise.

What is the truth? Who are we and what have we become or are we becoming? Zombies of the computer and whoever can manipulate it?

Do the headaches and dry eyes, other vision issues, irritability, rapid heart beats, excitement, secret feeling of being able to do things without being caught or having to face the consequence, sneezing, allergies, heightened anxiety about meeting deadlines and so on mean anything?

As computer users we probably never even think of all these things we suffer as anything. Why do we not take them seriously? Is our ability to exercise self-control and ability to know when something is wrong hampered?

These are some of the reasons why it may be necessary to find someone to be accountable to and why someone who can help keep a record of how we feel during computer use may be important to help us identify and deal with health issues before they set in.

What we cannot discern on our own may become clearer when we talk to someone who understands the issue.

Nobody knows all the toxic chemicals and minerals that computer use exposes humans to.

Some could have triggers and other functionalities that affect the fat breaking down process, metabolic rate, sugar, and carbohydrate and protein breakdown processes of the body.

There could also be those that make us crave all the wrong things such as processed foods and sodas.

Because computer use is addictive, (please refer to my book Computer Use Addiction and Withdrawal Syndromes: What You Need to Know for more details), we tend to spend more time than we need to on it

This is very significant in the issue of obesity in general and in the current national fight against childhood obesity.

If children are in an environment of adult computer use addictions, there is no one to exercise control. An adult that is out of control cannot effectively control a child's activity.

We will discuss more about this in the chapters that follow.

Please note that it is important to read this entire book carefully and also refer to my other books for more details on specific issues where indicated for complete understanding.

This is a short book meant to provide global information and so more details are provided in books that have been written to focus on the areas indicated to provide better clarity.

The heart and Information processing by the body
The heart is the master control or manager of the body that takes care of the other parts and meets the various nutritional needs of the different parts of the body by supplying nutrients all around via the bloodstream network.

It is an electrical organ and is the gateway to the human system. It controls the working of the brain and other organs to achieve the activity of motion and everything else that enable us to be moving beings on the earth.

It is the heart that receives the light from the sun that stimulates our ability to operate as humans. It is the heart that receives words (audible, inaudible words, thoughts and so on) and parses them and initiates the activity required by the words received.

Consequently, it is the heart that receives the artificial light that comes to us from the computer screen as well as the words and images we receive from the computer.

However, the way the heart normally receives information from natural light is not the same as it does from the computer as natural light contains stress handlers and controllers we call neurotransmitters that regulate the pace and intensity of receipt thereby avoiding damage.

The computer light however is artificial, has no life and consequently no handlers to manage the flow of information and light.

Consequently, over time our reserves of inhibitory neurotransmitters of handlers are depleted without replenishment by computer use activity.

This is why over time we could develop panic attacks, heart palpitations and so on as a result of overdose of electrical current from the computer coming to our hearts.

Any observant computer user will realize that computer use increases the heart rate. This is the reason why that happens.

In addition, the inhibitors that enable us self regulate, make wise choices and so on are heavily depleted in computer use as computer use involves continuous non stop mini and micro decision making. We are constantly making decisions while using the computer.

This depletion is why we get addicted and procrastinate on getting up from before it and easily lose our desire to exercise and move around when using the computer.

Thus computer use can exacerbate and even initiate the process of laziness and loss of desire for physical activities a recipe for weight gain and obesity.

Consequently, computer users need external prompting to make the decision to get up and move.

Computer use induced body Toxicity
There is also the issue of computer use induced body toxicity arising from the continual exposure to toxic artificial light and chemicals inherent in computer use.

These toxic lights and chemicals affect the body's ability to function as coded including the ability to perform proper digestive functions such as the ability to breakdown fats and sugars and so on that could lead to weight gain and obesity.

Oxygen depletion and excessive CO2 in computer use environment

Oxygen depletion affects the body's functions just as toxic light and chemicals do.

Operating computers generate a lot of CO2 (Carbon Dioxide) an action that depletes the availability of oxygen in the air. That is why some people may find it difficult to breath properly and deeply in a room full of computers.

When the body does not have enough oxygen to operate effectively all processes are affected.

Biochemical and Nutrient Depletion

Inherent in computer use are very harmful depletions of biochemials called neurotransmitter, hormones and so on some of which we discussed about earlier in this chapter.

Computer use unbeknown to many people also involves a heavy use of some certain minerals, vitamins and other nutrients and since people do not normally eat for computer use, they end up suffering the depletion of these nutrients and the resultant health consequences.

Even when tests by medical professionals show some of these depletions, they are unable to recognize the cause and consequently unnecessary medication resulting in new complications that never existed may set in.

The result is that whereas at the onset there was a situation that could easily be corrected, as a result of misdiagnosis and treatment we now have new issues without the first being resolved.

This is why we now have many health conditions that seem so stubborn and irresolvable. Situations that should never be medicated are being medicated because of the misguided approach that drugs are the solution to all issues.

Drugs actually never resolve anything. It is when patients realizing that they are ill and need to make some diet, exercise and other lifestyle changes such as resting and so on, make those changes, that there is a respite as coded systems cannot be resolved by medication but by falling in line with the code of operation of the system.

Our maker has given us a user manual we call the Bible or Scriptures, we will do well to follow it instead of trying to chart our own course to the ruin of our human machine.

Sleep Deprivation
Sleep deprivation as a result of computer use is especially prevalent in today's world, as Internet browsing, gaming and texting have become the norm for many people.

Depriving the body of much needed down time for self repair and maintenance is wrought with huge health issues including digestive and nutrient absorption issues which could result in weight gain, heart and other organ problems.

Please note that sleep deprivation is a self inflicted stress on the body with many unintended health consequence some of which could be life changing and even fatal in some cases.

The stress of obesity coupled with sleep deprivation could be a serious problem for the heart.

Computer Use addiction

As we have read in this book, computer use addiction is real and has become so commonplace it has become second nature to many people as our society has become computer use dependent for even simple things that really do not need computer use.

The allure of convenience has become a trap most people are unable to escape.

Abnormal Stress

The stresses that computer use places on our body's system are abnormal and very different to those we are coded to cope with.

That is because computer use is sedentary contrary to our normal coded way of exercising most of our body muscles in concert for most of life' activity.

In addition, we are exposed to artificially generated light and chemicals we are not coded with as well as various air moisture, ionization and other air and electrical imbalances not normal to us.

The abnormal nature of this stress means the body cannot readily cope with them and so they act as viruses and computer worms using up resources while damaging critical process paths essential for effective body functions.

Any weakened part in our system, for example if we are already overweight and procrastinate about physical activity, will be further deteriorated with resultant consequences. In this case obesity and if we are already obese, we find it difficult to do anything about it.

Chapter 5
Assisting Childhood Obesity Sufferers

According to a report in the Journal of the American Medical Association [5-1], some doctors are currently advocating that parents of children with life threatening obesity should lose custody of their kids to the state.

Before we take such draconian actions let us really think through what we are trying to achieve and see whether what we are advocating is really feasible or in the child's interest or whether we need a different approach.

I suppose the thinking is that if the children are placed with non obese people, then the problem will be solved.

Not so fast. It is not that simple. There is more than relationship involved here. These children know no one else but their parents who they trust. They will now be placed with strangers, who they do not know and who do not know them, in an environment that is strange.

They will now be battling many issues including a feeling of alienation, rejection, feeling a misfit, feeling of guilt towards their parents losing them and so on.

For children, having to battle all these psychological issues will obviously result in lifelong issues for these children.

Further, maybe there are some societal issues that are part of the issue and which may affect the children wherever they may be placed.

First off children are best off with their parents and should only be removed as a last ditch effort.

One of the reasons for obesity is the sedentary nature of the activities in the child's life.

As a society that is continually placing more and more emphasis on using technology to handle everything in life, we have set ourselves up for an obesity epidemic on a long-term basis.

That is because technology dependent activities are sedentary and a natural recipe for obesity.

As we have read in this book, Computer use involves the use of a few muscles leaving all others stationary. It is therefore sedentary in nature and may be a factor in weight gain for adults and kids.

It may also contribute to obesity because of the excessive production of cortisol from the unnatural stress of its use to our bodies.

Cortisol as we have read in chapter 2 is one of the known causes of obesity

When over time, parents lose their sense of self-control as a result of biochemical changes during computer use, they become unable to help their children establish control in the various aspects of their lives that are needed to control obesity.

One thing that many people fail to realize is that computer use inherently results in depletion of inhibitory neurotransmitters especially GABA and serotonin and the excessive release of excitatory ones which is why most people are addicted to its use and are unable to exercise self control in its use.

The National Center for Education Statistics in their statistical report on computer and internet use by students in 2003 [5-2] (based on information from the census bureau) said that "About 91percent (53 million persons) of children age 3 and over and in nursery school through grade 12 use computers, and about 59 percent (35 million persons) use the Internet.

The US Census bureau population survey [5-3], October 2009 meanwhile indicates that 76.7 percent of all households has someone with access to the Internet from a location.

Moving a child from one computer use based environment to another will not help if a child is already obese as the new parents will have the same problem as the old ones.

It may actually hurt the child more making him or her act out becoming a difficult child they never were before being placed into foster care.

For if the new parents or guardians or others in the household have computer use dependent jobs or are in any way heavily involved in the use of computer devices including laptops, desktops, notebooks, ipads, cell phones, blackberries, iphones, video games and so on, moving a child around may not achieve much or only achieve short term gains that are easily reversed.

A better approach may be to get the parents a lifestyle coach, social worker or relative who understands the computer use environment, what preventive measures to put in place and who also understands the biochemical issues involved in computer use, how these affect decision making and can therefore help both child and parents effect and maintain the changes needed, to work with them and their doctors.

It is a long hard road to establishing and maintaining self control when lost as a result of computer use exposure.

A coach, social worker or relative in the mix who they can be accountable to will give them someone who can take them by the hand through the long tough road in a way that helps them stick with the program.

If at all the child needs to be placed in foster care for some time, the foster parents too will need this help for the program to be successful.

If this is not done we may have temporary success that unravels pretty fast even before the child leaves foster care.

Consequently, having a policy of taking children from their parents may be counter productive without societal changes that ensure the change desired will really be accomplished.

Things are better done on a case-by-case basis using additional help as described above.

The effect on childhood obesity on the family
When anyone is obese in a family, the whole family is affected.

It means all have to watch what they eat, it curtails freedom and individual expression as everyone has to put the effect of their actions or words or activity on the obese person high up in the priority list before making decisions in an effort to help the obese family member.

When the obese person is a child, the need for care is doubled.

As we have read above, computer use is a recipe for weight gain. If parents are always on the computer, they are in danger of gaining weight from lack of activity making it difficult for them to exercise disciple with their children.

In addition, when too much time is spent on browsing and texting and games and so on there is a danger of the parents not getting adequate meals for their kids opting to get fast food or eat out rather than spending quality time cooking well balanced meals and paying close attention to their children's diet.

This to me is one of the reasons for the sharp rise in childhood obesity over the past few decades as computer use has become an epidemic and most people have become addicted to its use.

Consequently, not spending enough time monitoring children's diet and ensuring it is wholesome can be an unintended consequence of spending too much time using computerized tools and gadgets.

Other key healing tools things that could help include
1. Prayer. This is a fundamental and key healing tool.

2. Reading with the light of the sun – This will assist the body in producing more inhibitor reserves.

3. Strong support from family and friends

4. Avoid worry especially financial worries

5. Avoid other stresses

Chapter 6
More Obesity Trends Statistics

It is an open and well known secret that the U.S. is the most obese country in the world. We will start with U.S statistics and then move to global levels.

U.S National Trends

A paper by Katherine M. Flegal, PhD, Margaret D. Carroll, MSPH, Brian K. Kit, MD and Cynthia L. Ogden, PhD [6-1] detailing the result of a study on Prevalence of Obesity and Trends in the Distribution of Body Mass Index Among US Adults, 1999-2010, published in the journal of American Medical Association on January 17, 2012 has the following statistics:

1. Between 1980 and 1999, the prevalence of adult obesity (body mass index [BMI] ≥30) increased in the United States and the distribution of BMI changed. More recent data suggested a slowing or leveling off of these trends.

2. In 2009-2010 the age-adjusted mean BMI was 28.7 (95% CI, 28.3-29.1) for men and also 28.7 (95% CI, 28.4-29.0) for women. Median BMI was 27.8 (interquartile range [IQR], 24.7-31.7) for men and 27.3 (IQR, 23.3-32.7) for women. The age-adjusted prevalence of obesity was 35.7% (95% CI, 31.9%-39.2%) among adult men and 35.8% (95% CI, 34.0%-37.7%) among adult women.

3. Over the 12-year period from 1999 through 2010, obesity showed no significant increase among women overall (age- and race-adjusted annual change in odds

ratio [AOR], 1.01; 95% CI, 1.00-1.03; P= .07), but increases were statistically significant for non-Hispanic black women (P= .04) and Mexican American women (P= .046). For men, there was a significant linear trend (AOR, 1.04; 95% CI, 1.02-1.06; P< .001) over the 12-year period.

4. For both men and women, the most recent 2 years (2009-2010) did not differ significantly (P= .08 for men and P= .24 for women) from the previous 6 years (2003-2008). Trends in BMI were similar to obesity trends.

5. **Conclusion:** In 2009-2010, the prevalence of obesity was 35.5% among adult men and 35.8% among adult women, with no significant change compared with 2003-2008.

    The study on Trends over 5 Decades in U.S. Occupation-Related Physical Activity and Their Associations with obesity [2-1] that we looked at in chapter 2 has some interesting information.

    It said that the authors while acknowledging that the true causes of the obesity epidemic are not well understood and that there are few longitudinal population-based data published examining this issue, came to the following conclusion:

    'Over the last 50 years in the U.S. we estimate that daily occupation-related energy expenditure has decreased by more than 100 calories, and this reduction in energy expenditure accounts for a significant portion of the increase in mean U.S. body weights for men and women."

This atudy was conducted by by Timothy S. Church, Diana M. Thomas, Catrine Tudor-Locke, Peter T. Katzmarzyk, Conrad P. Earnest, Ruben Q. Rodarte, Corby K. Martin, Steven N. Blair, Claude Bouchard

The Centers for Disease Control and Prevention (CDC) has the following statistics [6-2]:

National trends
About one-third of U.S. adults (33.8%) are obese.
Approximately 17% (or 12.5 million) of children and adolescents aged 2—19 years are obese.
[Data from the National Health and Examination Survey (NHANES)]

Trend by States
1. During the past 20 years, there has been a dramatic increase in obesity in the United States and rates remain high.

2. In 2010, no state had a prevalence of obesity less than 20%.

3. Thirty-six states had a prevalence of 25% or more; 12 of these states (Alabama, Arkansas, Kentucky, Louisiana, Michigan, Mississippi, Missouri, Oklahoma, South Carolina, Tennessee, Texas, and West Virginia) had a prevalence of 30% or more.

Global Trends

According to the World Health Organization (WHO) [6-2], the mean BMI of the world's population increased dramatically between 1980 and 2008.

Globally, around 35% of adults aged 20 and over were overweight in 2008, while around 12% of adults aged 20 and over were obese.

According to the WHO mean Body Mass Index article [1-3] referred to in chapter 1,

1   In 2008, 35% of adults aged 20+ were overweight (BMI $\geq$ 25 kg/m2) (34% men and 35% of women).

2   The worldwide prevalence of obesity more than doubled between 1980 and 2008. In 2008, 10% of men and 14% of women in the world were obese (BMI $\geq$30 kg/m2), compared with 5% for men and 8% for women in 1980.

3   An estimated 205 million men and 297 million women over the age of 20 were obese a total of more than half a billion adults worldwide.

4   Worldwide, at least 2.8 million people die each year as a result of being overweight or obese,

5   An estimated 35.8 million (2.3%) of global DALYs (Disability Adjusted Life Years) are caused by overweight or obesity.

6   Overweight and obesity lead to adverse metabolic effects on blood pressure, cholesterol, triglycerides and insulin resistance.

7   Risks of coronary heart disease, ischemic stroke and
     type 2 diabetes mellitus increase steadily with
     increasing body mass index (BMI), a measure of
     weight relative to height.

8   Raised body mass index also increases the risk of
     cancer of the breast, colon, prostate, endometrium,
     kidney and gall bladder.

9   Mortality rates increase with increasing degrees of
     overweight, as measured by body mass index.

10   To achieve optimum health, the median body mass
     index for an adult population should be in the range of
     21 to 23 kg/m2, while the goal for individuals should
     be to maintain body mass index in the range 18.5 to
     24.9 kg/m2.

11   There is increased risk of co-morbidities for body mass
     index 25.0 to 29.9, and moderate to severe risk of co-
     morbidities for body mass index greater than 30.

Chapter 7
More Suggested Practical Solutions

In addition to the various solutions discussed under each chapter, here are some more suggested practical solutions:

Have a computer free day once a week
The essence is to get away from both the toxic environment and allow the body to heal as well as get away from the sedentary weight gain prone activity called computer use.

Do not replace computer free time with television watching. Spend the time in exercise and other energy consuming activities such as real book reading, gardening, house cleaning, making real home made meals and so on.

Remember that video games and cell phones are computers too and avoid sitting in one spot all day calling all your friends and sending text messages.

Take computer free vacations
It is important that we give our bodies rest time away from toxic exposure to enhance its ability to self repair. Taking a computer free vacation at least once a year would certainly go a long way in achieving this objective.

Establish daily Computer Use timeouts
Establish a daily computer use timeout throughout the day and especially at night. Use no computer devise during that time but only carry out functions that are natural to the body's way of operation. For example read only physical books during these times, get up and pick up things with your hand, talk to people face to face and so on.

Take a weekly day of rest

According to the user manual, the human body is programmed to take rests and a day of rest is required once a week for optimal performance.

Our maker set this example for us by taking a day of rest at the beginning. Even the earth takes its period of rest and the best way to cultivate the land for bumper harvest that is truly healthy is to allow a year of rest after every seven year to allow the ground to heal and replenish so the crops we harvest can produce the nutrients we need in the right grade and quantity.

In my case my day of rest is Saturday the Sabbath of our maker, following his instructions to my forefathers when they implored him to stay with them. They wanted his presence in their midst.

He gave them the law to show them what they needed to do to be able to stay in his presence without being destroyed by his holiness.

He gave them this instruction for their safety, showing them how to operate their systems for optimal production.

That is why the principle of taking a day of rest is important. It is the way we are coded to operate and like any other computer system, operating without rest period will breakdown the system as the maintenance process becomes overloaded.

Small wonder our food is now one of the greatest sources of toxic pollution in our body system and we no longer get the nutrients we are supposed to from taking our food.

Taking rest time also reduces stress and avoids overproduction of cortisol.

Diet
It is common knowledge that we are what we eat. Consequently, eating for example foods devoid of adequate fiber or those that are filled with sugar will be a problem.

While processed sugar is harmful, taking natural sweet foods like fruits when in their natural forms without human intervention such as genetic modification is very healthy as the foods get naturally processed by the human system according to the code without unprocessed leftovers that act like viruses and malware in the system.

Avoid processed and genetically modified foods. They are not compatible with the human body process, will not be fully processed and also actually contain toxic chemicals that many a times result in the inability of the body to breakdown the food resulting in fat deposits.

It is extremely important that you avoid other sources of toxin if you are a computer user. Your diet should be as toxin free as possible.

Go for daily walks
A look at the words of our user manual and even the most casual observation of one's own life and that of others around shows us we were designed to do a lot of walking.

Consequently, daily walks are a necessity for optimal body function. Walk as much as you can. As you walk, the body processes the light fields or biochemical/neurotransmitters in sunlight building up resources.

Since walking is our natural mode of exercise we get the perfect advantage from exercising from it.

The most important thing is consistency. Hence, the advocacy in this book for daily walks.

As you burn up the fat and reduce your weight you will feel better in every area of your life.

You will also find computer use less stressful as you build up reserves of inhibitory neurotransmitters while walking that can be released during computer use later.

Let the fresh air in
According to the user manual, we see that man was made to be an outdoor person, That is because his life is coded into him from the sun and he gets his oxygen from the atmosphere.

The rain powers the growth of his food and he was made to take care of the earth for his maker.

Consequently when we shut out the outdoors we create a less than optimal environment for living, which affects the various processes in our system.

That is why lack of outdoor activity wreaks so much havoc in people including mental, digestive and so on during the cold months of winter.

Let the sunlight in when using the computer
It is important to let sunlight in when using the computer since computer light is artificial and cannot stimulate our brains to produce neurotransmitters. Computer use uses up a lot of our inhibitory neurotransmitter required in the presence of light.

Exercise during computer use
There are discreet exercises one can do during computer use to ensure one uses as many muscles as possible.

Have healthy familial relationships
This is a critical support you need. If you are giving support please be sincere. Do not pamper the person you are supporting. Lovingly speak to them but be firm

Make a conscious effort to be more active outdoors
Remember this and make it one of your daily goals.

Take Breaks while working
Taking breaks while working ensures more movement of muscles and body parts creating a healthier body. It also provides regular breaks from the toxic addictive environment of computer use providing an opportunity to exercise self control.

Virtual Entrapment
More and more people are becoming entrapped in virtual worlds of their own making becoming more and more unable to handle the realities of the real world as they spend more time in the virtual than in the real one.

This is an avoidable recipe for relational, behavioral and mental issues. However once in this trap it is very difficult to get out. It is not an issue that is easily recognized by the virtualized person and if and when they do realize there is a problem, they are unable to figure their way out.

They need help. The issue is a biochemical problem and trying to reason them out of it will not work. It has to be dealt on a biochemical level in a holistic way. This takes a long time and I am talking about years of consistent lifestyle change.

Accountability
If possible, find someone to be accountable to for keeping to computer timeouts and other self imposed computer use limits.

Set fixed daily computer use time
This will help to reduce the addiction tendency inherent in computer use and encourage body movement since the whole day is not spent in front of the computer.

Avoid filling the void with television. Spend the time helping your body rest from exposure to artificial light. If you need to read, read real books

It will also help to reduce computer use induced stress and laziness that sets in from over indulgence in sedentary activities such as computer use.

Avoid exotic websites
Many people get caught in exotic websites many of which could be dangerous and lead to a tendency to want to indulge in those activities presented when back in the real world.

Such websites include pornographic sites, adult websites, gambling and so on.

Such sites are set up with a play on light combinations to get people hooked the first time with a high that brings them back.

That is why it is dangerous to visit them even once.

They are very addictive as the lights have a high level of intensity that forces the body to use up more inhibitory neurotransmitters resulting in over firing of excitatory ones which is the high that people feel when at these sites.

Unknown to them they are creating untold damage in their body's system that can lead to many strange health issues that would be difficult for doctors to diagnose.

Do not use the computer for leisure

Many people seem to think a dangerous tool like the computer is a tool that can be used for leisure. The truth is that it is not a tool for leisure. It should be used as necessary Not to while away the time.

Parents do not place your children in front of the computer to keep him or her quiet. They will become addicted and their developing brains cannot handle the high level of toxicity inherent in computer use.

What may seem harmless may result in a lifetime of mental and/or behavioral issues down the road or even in debilitating diseases not normally associated with computer use and that could easily be misdiagnosed as resulting from something else.

Acknowledge your over dependency on computer use

When people think about computers they only think about the laptop and desktop. They forget to acknowledge the various other devices we take for granted as essential items in our lives that are actually computers.

In fact, anything that has a screen emitting artificial light and that has something you can type on to control what you see on the screen with or that can be controlled automatically is a computerized device.

When there is a screen it is more harmful but the motorized auto control and auto pilot devices are harmful too as they emit toxic chemicals from the artificial electromagnetic fields (i.e. artificially generated light fields) operating in them (an example is a microwave oven).

They all have mini and micro computer chips in them that power them). They all have the same health effects as the toxic electrical fields that come off the desktop's Central Processing Unit (CPU).

The television has no keyboard but has all the other computer component and is also a computer devise. If you open up the back of your television it has a motherboard that compares to that of a laptop i.e. mainly wires and magnets.

We can all see now why this issue is affecting our health and creating a lot of confusion in our body's system. We are all over exposed. When we add the artificial light we use to see in our homes, offices and schools we have a recipe for health related problems that the medical profession is not equipped to handle and that drugs cannot resolve.

That is because the problem is happening at the soul level of our being that cannot be medicated and that is responsible for managing, operating and repairing the physical part of us that we can see and touch.

These final two solutions should only be done under the supervision of a medical professional.
1. Detoxification
2. Fasting

Chapter 8
Why it is so hard to Change Behavior

Getting and using information about preventive measures to take as a computer user is not easy and here is why

There are real biochemical complications that take place in our systems that make it difficult for computer users to stop procrastinating and face the reality of the health effect their activity is having on them.

Human behavior is dependent on the balance of light fields (biochemicals) we call neurotransmitters in the brain. The decision with regards to behavior that the heart takes at anytime depends on the availability of these resources for carrying out the action required.

Consequently, a person may intellectually know he or she needs to be more active but may not have enough resources to even fully understand the import of this knowledge and would therefore not process its effect on his or her health effectively to take action.

In some cases, the import is known but the neurotransmitters responsible for actually taking the decision to act may be depleted or the ones responsible for understanding what needs to be done may be. In some other cases, the inhibitors needed to stop procrastinating may be depleted.

These are inhibitors (control) neurotransmitters that enable a person appreciate the urgency of a needed action.

During computer use, the neurotransmitters that get depleted first are the inhibitors. They depend on access to sunlight.

We receive light fields from the sun that are converted from those needed in a static body like the sun that is totally self controlled rising and setting on cue without stop no matter what into that which is needed in human bodies that require motion.

When we receive these neurotransmitters, they are converted by our natural coded process in a reaction with amino acids and other required nutrients into the variation of inhibitors required for the human body.

Natural light is life containing which is what enables us to live. Artificially generated light is lifeless and so has no neurotransmitters and cannot stimulate their production.

Consequently when in the computer use environment whether it is the laptop or desktop or cell phone or video games or a picture only without typing system as with the television, we are continually using up our resources without the automatic replacement needed for proper body system function.

That depletion is why we are reluctant to get off the computer even when we know we should. It is what gives rise to computer use addiction.

It is cumulative and so the more computer use we have, the more we procrastinate and lose control and even fail to understand the full health impact of what we are doing. We seem unable to control ourselves.

That is because our control mechanism has become impaired.

This is why gamers for example seem so stubborn and carefree and inhibited.

It is because the sense of danger is lost. The ability to recognize danger, discretion and so on is heavily depleted and consequently danger has to actually be experience before being recognized.

Note To The Reader:

About the author:

Adetutu Ijose, is a technology and accounting professional with over 25 years of intensive computer use exposure who suffered life threatening computer related health conditions the doctors could neither diagnose not treat.

In desperation and with a good knowledge of codes and how they work, she studied the human computer user manual we call the Bible until she was able to understand why and how the computer hurts our body's system as well as the preventive and repair kits placed in nature by our maker.

She also began to realize that many issues not normally attributable to computer use were actually due to or exacerbated by computer use.

One of those issues is obesity, a condition primarily based on underutilization of body muscles coupled with poor diet – 2 issues that computer users are very guilty of.

After reading about the new wave of children being taken from their parents as a result of being obese, she realized she needed to bring what she knew to the table in addressing the obesity epidemic as computer use was not being discussed or even acknowledge in the debate on the issue.

Knowing that our modern lifestyle of heavy computer use was contributory to the problem, she realized that it was important to make the information she had public in a bid to help everyone.

She is now passing on her understanding about computer use induced issues through her many books, other writings and speaking activities so others can receive help.

Adetutu Ijose is a speaker on the subject of computer use induced health conditions. She is also a contributor to several online article websites and blogs including content sites associatedcontent.com and examiner.com. She has also been interviewed on radio.

To schedule a speaking or consulting engagement, interview, so on with the author, please contact Adetutu Ijose at http://www.foodsthathealdaily.com.

For Adetutu Ijose's online press kit or for press releases and other media matters and inquiries, please go to http://lessosilearnedthehardway.com/AdetutuIjoseMediaPre ssKit.aspx

Discover other titles by Adetutu Ijose to help you better understand responsible computer use and how computer use affect us all as well as what we need to do to prevent and manage these issues at www.foodsthathealydaily.com, www.amazon.com and other online stores. Ebook versions of this and other books by Adetutu Ijose are available at amazon.com, Barnes and Nobles, Smashword.com and other ebook stores. A complete list is provided below.

Email Adetutu Ijose at adetutuijose@gmail.com or computerblessings@gmail.com

Connect with Adetutu Ijose Online:
Facebook: http://www.facebook.com/home.php

Computer Use Induced Health Conditions related books by Adetutu Ijose as at the time of writing are:

1) *Lessons I Learned the Hard Way: How to Identify, Minimize, Treat and Manage Computer Related Health Condition*

2) *Computer Related Health Condition: Understanding the Human Computer*

3) *Healing Juicing Smoothie and Milk Shake Recipes: Juices, Smoothies and Milk Shakes that Help the Body Achieve its Self Healing Process*

4) *Healing Meals Recipe: Meals that Help the Body Achieve its Self Healing Process*

5) *Cyber Bullying: How and Why Bullies operate*

6) *Global Epidemic: The Human Abuse of the Computer*

7) *Computer Use Addiction and Withdrawal Syndromes: What You Need to Know*

8) *Teenage and Adult Texting Addictions: What You Need to Know*

9) *Allergies, Asthma and Computer Use: The Contributory Effects of Computer Use to Allergies and Asthma Trends*

10) *Computer Use Induced Stress: What You Need to Know*

11) *The Health effect of Video Games: What You Need to Know*

12) *Eyes, Vision and Computer Use: How You can Protect Yourself From Technology Use Induced Harm*

13) *Obesity and Computer Use: What You Need to Know*

For other titles published after this book – Obesity and Computer Use, please go to amazon.com and other online stores or visit my website www.foodsthathealdaily.com

References

1-1 National Library of Medicine – Pubmed Health
http://www.ncbi.nlm.nih.gov/pubmedhealth/PMH0004
552/

1-2 WHO Child Growth Standards Report – Executive
Summary
http://www.who.int/childgrowth/standards/tr_summary
/en/

1-3 National Institute of Health (NIH MEDPLUS) article
on How To Know Your Body Mass Index (BMI)
http://www.nlm.nih.gov/medlineplus/magazine/issues/
winter07/articles/winter07pg16.html

1-4 WHO article on Mean Body Max Index (BMI)
http://www.who.int/gho/ncd/risk_factors/bmi_text/en/i
ndex.html

2-1 Michelle Obama's Let's Move Initiative
http://www.letsmove.gov/

2-2 study on Trends over 5 Decades in U.S. Occupation-
Related Physical Activity and Their Associations with
obesity by Timothy S. Church, Diana M. Thomas, Catrine
Tudor-Locke, Peter T. Katzmarzyk, Conrad P. Earnest,
Ruben Q. Rodarte, Corby K. Martin, Steven N. Blair,
Claude Bouchard
http://www.plosone.org/article/info%3Adoi%2F10.1371%2
Fjournal.pone.0019657

2-3 International Journal of Obesity research on the link
between obesity and cotisol -

http://www.nature.com/ijo/journal/v28/n9/full/0802715a.ht
ml

3-1 Mayo Clinic Childhood Obesity
http://www.mayoclinic.com/health/childhood-
obesity/DS00698

3-2 WEBMED article on Obesity in Children
http://children.webmd.com/obesity-children

3-3 WHO Growth Reference – BMI ages 5-19
http://www.who.int/growthref/who2007_bmi_for_age/en/

3-4 WHO Report on the Development of new Child
Growth Standards -
http://www.who.int/childgrowth/1_what.pdf

3-5 WHO Report on Development of a WHO growth
reference for school-aged children and adolescents
http://www.who.int/growthref/growthref_who_bull/en/inde
x.html

4-1 News Release dated 25 May 2011 from the Pennington
Biomedical Research Center on the obesity epidemic
http://www.prnewswire.com/news-releases/pennington-
biomedical-research-center-study-suggests-decreases-in-u-
s-occupation-energy-levels-a-significant-trigger-of-obesity-
epidemic-122614203.html,

5-1 JAMA journal commentary on state intervention in life
threatening childhood obesity - http://jama.ama-
assn.org/content/306/2/206.full

5-2 NCES data in computer and internet use by students -
http://nces.ed.gov/pubs2006/2006065.pdf

5-3 Download the U.S. Census bureau statistics on "Internet use in the United States" from http://www.census.gov/population/www/socdemo/computer/2009.html

6-1 Paper by Katherine M. Flegal, PhD, Margaret D. Carroll, MSPH, Brian K. Kit, MD and Cynthia L. Ogden, PhD 4-1 detailing the result of a study on Prevalence of Obesity and Trends in the Distribution of Body Mass Index Among US Adults, 1999-2010, published in the journal of American Medical Association on January 17, 2012 http://jama.ama-assn.org/content/early/2012/01/11/jama.2012.39.full

6-2 CDC obesity data trends trends by state http://www.cdc.gov/obesity/data/trends.html

6-3 WHO article on Overweight and Obesity http://www.who.int/gho/ncd/risk_factors/overweight/en/

INDEX

A

F

Food, 15, 16, 18, 34, 41, 42, 43

G

Global, 18, 25, 35, 38, 53

H

Heart, 11,19, 23, 25, 26, 28, 39, 48

I

Inhibitors, 26, 48, 49
Inhibitory, 26, 31, 43, 45
Internet, 22, 23, 28, 32
Iphones, 22, 32

L

Lifestyles, 15, 17
light, 7, 18, 25, 26, 27, 29, 34, 42, 43, 45, 46, 47, 48, 49
Lives, 17, 23, 31, 46

M

Maker, 28, 41, 43, 51
Medication, 7, 27, 28
Muscles, 29, 31, 44, 51

N

Neurotransmitter, 15, 17, 42
Neurotransmitters, 25, 26, 31, 42, 43, 46, 48, 49

O

obesity, 5, 10, 12, 13, 14, 15, 16, 17, 18, 19, 20, 22, 24, 26, 27,
    28, 29, 30, 31, 33, 34, 35, 36, 37, 38, 51, 54
Overweight, 10, 12, 13, 20, 29, 38, 39